D1563910

RISE UP

Defining Your Cancer Journey, So Cancer Doesn't Define You

By

Bridgette Alpha Akins

This book is dedicated to:

The Living God who surrounds me with grace, mercy and love and provides me with the wisdom to be strong and courageous.

Matt, Jack Matthew and Evangeline for always filling my days with love and laughter. I love you more than anything in this world!

Table of Contents

Introduction

Love and Laughter are two words that I have always used to guide my intentions and actions but on March 18, 2020 those are not the words that filled my mind or my heart. This is the day that everything went from just another day to the scariest day of my life. In this book, I share my story of battling cancer during quarantine and the coronavirus. I detail my fears, tears, joy, and strength. I also share action steps that will allow you to face life's biggest challenges with clarity, confidence, peace, and positivity. As a certified health and life coach, I have personally used these practices to bring calmness and clarity to my life especially during my cancer diagnosis and journey. I have worked with clients guiding them through the same action steps to find purpose and achieve their goals. In this book, we explore ways to

- Acknowledge, Accept and Name Challenges
- Recognize a Higher Power

- Identify Support Systems
- Uncover Your MoFa (Motivating Factor)
- Set and Achieve Goals
- Gain Confidence
- Embrace Gratitude and much more.

Throughout the book, you will also discover W.O.W. moments: Words of Wisdom, and Words of Wellness. These were inspired by the philosophy of nurturing the whole self. A philosophy that I have adopted in my own life. W.O.W. moments can be explained as follows.

Words of Wisdom:

These are blog entries or excerpts from my own journaling that spoke to me or held significance during my journey.

Words of Wellness:

Strategies or activities that I used throughout my journey to nourish my mind, body and soul.

Cancer was a journey much like that of everyday life.

It was filled with highs, lows, faith, fear, joy, vulnerability, strength, humility and love. It was through this journey that I was able to look at my life in the rawest form and evaluate my priorities and habits. Using the practices outlined in this book I was motivated to fight through the toughest days and cherish the best days. I challenge you to use this book in the same way.

Are you ready to RISE UP?

Then Ready, Set, Read!

Love and Laughter,

Bridgette

PART I: Life Changes: What To Do When It Does

"Ain't it funny how life changes
You wake up, ain't nothing the same
and life changes
You can't stop it, just hop on the train and
You never know what's gonna happen"
-Thomas Rhett

January in the Capital District of New York started the same as any other year...cold! Although my southern roots are often chilled during this season, I have come to appreciate the snow and stillness of the winter months. Although 2020 started as expected, most of us could not have imagined the changes that were about to take place and impact everyone across the nation and the world.

In our home, there was yet another impactful change

coming our way. I have always embraced change, and appreciated the present, but with so many things happening in the world around us, I wasn't ready for what was coming my way. Life doesn't wait for us to be ready for change, it just presents itself, and it is up to us how we handle it.

I had spent the last few years focused on being healthy, being in tune with my body, running a half marathon and practicing yoga to help me stay connected, so when I began to feel strangely fatigued and ill, I knew something was wrong. I tried to chalk it up to it being winter, as I typically tried to be more in tune with the circadian rhythms. I don't work out as often or with as much intensity, I eat heartily and adjust my sleep habits to better reflect the timing of the day. I tried to justify the symptoms but in the end I knew I had to listen to my body.

It was March 13th that my husband, Matt, said we should take a long weekend so that I could unwind, relax, take it easy and maybe feel better. I spent the weekend feeling lethargic, bloated, restless and in pain. I wasn't getting better. When my sister in law, Alesha,who is a physician's assistant for an OBGYN, suggested that I be seen on Monday the 16th, we had no idea what was coming and that our lives would never be the same.

Chapter One: Just Breathe

"Breathing In, I calm my body and mind. Breathing out, I smile. Dwelling in the present moment I know that this is the only moment."

-Thich Nhat Hanh

After spending the weekend feeling like I was getting worse, and then making it to the appointment on Monday the 16th, I was sent to a specialist on Wednesday the 18th. While I had no family history or precursors, the OBGYN, Dr. H., felt that the ovarian cyst I had developed should be tested, just to be safe. It was a two and a half-hour drive to Plattsburgh to see the specialist, Dr. E. The long trip added to the exhaustion and worry of this quickly unfolding diagnosis. Dr. E. did an ultrasound himself and said, "This is probably cancer, we need to get it out now." Two days later, on Friday the 20th he scheduled the surgery. To go from just a cyst to cancer in less than a week was very shocking for all of us. I think somewhere deep down I knew it was a possibility. I'd used WebMD and I'd Googled some of the symptoms and knew that it was a possibility but nobody seemed to think that was going to be what this was. The hardest thing for me was looking at Matt when the doctor said that I had cancer.

The news was a shock and all that lie ahead seemed unimaginable. However, the hardest thing for me was to see my husband, the rock of our family and the man who loves me unconditionally be brought to tears. He was shocked and devastated and trying to hold it together. I knew this cancer journey was going to be hard not only for me but for the entire family.

I got a call, Thursday afternoon, regarding the surgery that the governor had changed regulations and that I'd have to go by myself. Matt couldn't come with me. We drove the two and a half hours to Plattsburgh once again. He had to drop me off and I had to go in by myself. I knew this was going to be difficult but I couldn't have imagined just how difficult. We arrived at the hospital early and had time to chat and pray. Praying that the surgery went well, that the news would be the best it could be and that God would calm and protect us all. The time had come for me to go in. We drove to the door, shed many tears and gave our final hugs and kisses. For a person that is not usually very emotional, I was a mess. Tears, sobbing, shortness of breath, my body was experiencing so many emotions. The surgery got delayed because of different things, and my husband had to spend all day walking around, sitting in the car, worried and waiting.

The next three hours were extremely easy for me because I was unconscious. I can't fathom what it was like for Matt to be alone just waiting for an update. He was also tasked with delivering the news to others, the most difficult being my parents and his. Of course, the most difficult conversation would be with our children but that would be face to face at a later time. Just as I couldn't fathom what it was like for my husband to take all of this in, I also couldn't imagine how it felt for my parents to be almost 1,000 miles away and hear the news that their baby girl had cancer. The news was going to be hard for all of our family and friends. So, in those few hours, I was the lucky one.

When I finally awoke in recovery, I was greeted by a smiling nurse holding an orchid and card delivered by my amazing husband. I later found out that he walked around the town of Plattsburgh in search of a store that hadn't been closed due to the pandemic to find the gift. Once he found the store and gift the skies opened and the rain began to fall and he had to walk three miles back to the hospital with this delicate orchid. I believe God knew how hard he tried and how much I needed to see that gift when I awoke because it was undamaged by the rain and it was beautiful.

During surgery, the doctor removed the cyst that was fourteen centimeters at the time and drained three and a half liters of fluid. This definitely explained why I looked and felt like I was pregnant. We knew going in that if it was cancerous, I would need a hysterectomy. I knew it was the case as soon as the nurses came in to take care of me. I also knew the worst was yet to come.

I spent the next days and weeks recovering from surgery. With thirty-two staples from the bottom of my belly button through my c-section scar to my pubic bone, I was a little sore to say the least but I felt so much better than before. Each day my body became stronger and I was starting to feel myself again. I was walking every day, helping build a tepee and even using the chainsaw. It was very empowering! I was feeling great but in the back of my mind, I knew this was only temporary and that my body was about to take a blow like nothing it had ever felt before. Five weeks out from surgery I would begin chemotherapy.

The year had presented so many changes already. And this was only the beginning. It would be 13 weeks of being there and we had only packed for a long weekend.

Words of Wisdom – Just Breathe

Apr 18, 2020

Written By Bridgette Akins

As I sit today and write this post I think about how much has changed for all of us. I have been working for months on the content I wanted to share and the design of my new website. I was almost ready to go live and then life as we know it was sent into a whirlwind. COVID19, coronavirus and social distancing have become a part of our everyday vocabulary. Working and learning from home have become a new norm for most.

Amidst all of this it has also been a time of personal change. Last year at this time I was celebrating my birthday by running a half marathon. This year I am tackling a different challenge for my birthday - cancer. I was diagnosed with ovarian cancer after experiencing symptoms for only a couple of weeks and otherwise being healthy. As I contemplate my first chemotherapy treatment it is just another reminder of how quickly things can change. Today I am sharing the things I do to stay calm and find peace during uncertain times.

Breathe

I use a 5-5-7 breath. Simply inhale for 5 seconds, hold the breath for 5 seconds and exhale for 7 seconds. This will allow your mind and body to relax.

Ritual - On days that I find the most difficult I have a few ritualistic things that I do.

Shower

Listen to motivating or uplifting songs. My current go to is More Than Anything by Amy Grant.

Get dressed in clothes that make you feel good.

Journal

Just write it all down. It is amazing how therapeutic it can be just to get your thoughts out of your head and on to paper. I like to use pens in different colors.

It seems to make even the most mundane thoughts joyful.

Prayer and Meditation

Whether you pray, meditate or do both find a way to connect to that which is greater than you. For me prayer offers a level of honesty, peace and comfort that I don't find in anything else.

Get Outside

Fresh air and sunshine are good for the body, mind and soul. Even if it is only a walk to the mailbox make sure you take time to get outside each day and use your senses to take in the beauty of nature.

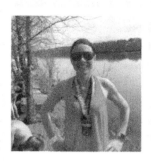

APRIL 2019
HALF MARATHON

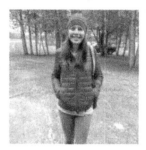

APRIL 2020
DIAGNOSED
WITH CANCER

Words of Wellness – 5-5-7 Breathing

With all that was changing around me I found this to be an exercise vital to me being able to focus and calm my body and mind. I love it because it can be done anywhere at any time. All you need to do is focus on relaxing and how it makes your body feel.

Just as the title states you will inhale for 5 seconds, hold the breath for 5 seconds and then exhale for 7 seconds. The exhale should be a little longer than the inhale.

Begin in a comfortable position.
Close your eyes if you prefer.

Inhale – 1,2,3,4,5
Hold - 5,4,3,2,1
Exhale – 7,6,5,4,3,2,1
Become conscious of your breathing.

Notice the rise and fall of your chest and stomach.

Tune in to your heightened awareness.

What do you notice?

How do you feel?

Repeat 10x

Chapter Two: Cancer Has a Definition but It Doesn't Define You

"In the midst of winter I finally learned that there lived in me an invincible summer."

Albert Camus

It was only March, but the year had already given me more than I wanted to handle. Not just me, but my family as well. There was so much to endure, and so much to learn, but one of the things that was therapeutic for me was the song from Natalie Grant called *More Than Anything,* which became my fight song. When I was in pain or just overwhelmed, I would take a bath, I would listen to this song, and I would just cry. I embraced and acknowledged my emotions, the pain that I felt, and I let it go. I just prayed, "God, this is yours, not mine. I can't do anything with it. I can't fix this. This is how I feel. I am physically, emotionally, mentally done."

I don't think there was ever a time that I thought I was going to give up because there were so many important things that were worth fighting for. My kids, my husband, so many other things driving me. But, there were low times. There was even a time where I just thought, I don't know if I can take anymore. After crying and praying, I would get out of the bathtub and say to myself, "Okay, we're doing this. We're still doing this."

It was definitely a gradual experience. I started journaling. I wrote the whole story from the beginning. Matt bought me a journal and I wrote in it every day. I wrote just whether it was how I felt, what I did or what I ate. I felt like I needed to chronicle my journey.

Defining my cancer journey, so it didn't define me, was part of my healing. In my appointments, in my surgery, my follow-ups, I heard a lot of, "Oh you have cancer and this is what's going to happen". It was a long list of side effects and what to expect. I did experience them but I couldn't let these circumstances dictate who I was or what I was. In a burst of strength, I said to myself, "Okay, I have cancer. Here's what the research shows me. Here's what the doctors tell me. But this is my journey, so what am I going to do to define it for myself?"

Being a health coach and life coach, I kept telling myself, "Okay, I can do this." Practice what you preach, right? It was meant to be therapeutic for me to start writing, but before too long, other people reached out to me and said, "I've been following your blog and it's really great when I have these days where I feel low, it helps me tell myself "Okay, I can do this" or "This is such an inspirational story and your positivity really helps." It became motivation for me. Not only was I helping myself through something very difficult, but I am helping people that are struggling in their own way, just by writing it down.

Words of Wisdom – Let's Talk About Your O's

Important Info About Ovarian Cancer

(Information from www.OvarianCancerProject.org)

Symptoms & Risks

Let's talk about your O's -as in your ovaries. Ovarian cancer is the most fatal gynecological disease, and with no screening test, knowing the symptoms and risk factors can save your life. So, if you experience any of the following for more than two weeks, it's time to speak up!

Bloating
Pelvic or abdominal pain
Difficulty eating or feeling full quickly
Urinary symptoms (Urgency or frequency)

Risk Factors for Ovarian Cancer

Age: Your risk increases with your age, most women with Ovarian Cancer are diagnosed over the age of 55.

Family History: Your risk is higher if you have a close blood relative, who has had breast cancer prior to age 50, ovarian cancer at any age, or male breast cancer at any age.

Personal History: Women who have had cancer of the breast, uterus, colon or rectum have a higher risk of ovarian cancer.

Reproductive History: If you have never had children or have a history of difficulty getting pregnant, you are at increased risk.

Hormone Replacement Therapy: If you have taken Hormone Replacement Therapy, you may be at higher risk.

Ethnicity: White women from European and North America have a higher risk, as do Jewish women of Eastern European (Ashkenazi) descent.

Endometriosis: If you have had a history of endometriosis, you are at higher risk of ovarian cancer.

Genetic Testing: Genetic testing indicating you have BRCA 1 or 2, or Lynch Syndrome also known as HNPCC puts you at a much higher risk for ovarian cancer.

Obesity: Being obese can put you at higher risk for some types of ovarian cancer.

Disclaimer: The information above is designed to aid women in making decisions about appropriate gynecologic care and does not substitute for evaluations with qualified medical professionals familiar with you.

Words of Wellness – Brain Dump

On a blank sheet or scrap paper list any thoughts and feelings that are currently cluttering your brain.

Take 5 minutes and scribble down whatever thoughts and emotions pop up.

Once you have completed the exercise throw out the paper (remember to recycle :)

Releasing these thoughts and emotions will make room for you to focus on your journey and conquer this challenge.

Journaling

No matter what your journey it is yours and it deserves to be told. Find a notebook or invest in an actual journal. Whichever you choose, be sure to chronicle your experience.

For your first journal entry find a spot outdoors to sit and observe.

Using all 5 senses notice what is around you.

After spending a few minutes observing with your senses begin to practice your 5-5-7 breathing.

Once you have completed 5 rounds of breathing take out your journal and pen and write, scribble or draw about how you feel.

If you don't have a journal handy feel free to use the space below.

PART II: Be Strong, Be Kind, Be Beautiful and Make a Plan

"Don't be pushed around by the fears in your mind.
Be led by the dreams in your heart."
Roy T. Bennett

I knew I had to start setting goals. My goal became a mantra, "Be positive." After all, that was my goal with this whole journey. Whatever I did, I needed to be positive. That didn't mean that I didn't cry and go through excruciating pain. It meant that once I embraced that and eventually let it go, that I could find the positivity in every day.

I knew without a doubt that I had to form a plan. I had to give myself grace, and when I felt like I couldn't do it anymore, or I couldn't stick to a healthy diet because I just wanted to have a chocolate milkshake, that it was okay because that is what I needed at that moment. I had to ask for help, I had to embrace the good, the bad, the pain, and the changes, along with my bald head. So what was this plan? What did I need to map out? I needed to know what I was facing, and create the goals I needed to achieve.

My plan included finding ways to embrace and release the emotions, having goals and finding those anchors that were a reminder of the goals—for me it was a song. It was having a routine. Learning things to calm my body like certain breathing exercises, certain meditations, and then having those statements that you really believe, "I'm strong." "I can do this." "I'm a fighter." Those are ways to mentally, emotionally get yourself in the right place so then physically you can deal with all that's about to come.

Chapter Three: Be Still and Know

"Be still and know that I am God."

Psalm 46:10

I was five weeks post-surgery and it was time for my first treatment. I started the day with what had become my daily ritual. I would soak in a hot bath while listening to and singing my fight song – More Than Anything by Natalie Grant-, cry and pray. I was overwhelmed by what was happening but I was always put at ease after this routine knowing that God heard me and that no matter what lies ahead that God had always gone before me and prepared the way and this time would be no different. All I needed was faith and that is something I already had.

My treatment was by all accounts uneventful. I spent the hours of time dozing in and out as the medicine made me quite groggy. I ate a few snacks but didn't find myself very hungry. Other than doze I spent most of the time walking to the bathroom. As a teacher who is used to scheduling bathroom breaks around lunch or specials it blew my mind that a person could actually go to the restroom ten times in a six-hour window. If you're a teacher you know what I'm talking about. I tried to write in my journal but I was so sleepy my handwriting started to turn into scribbles. I look at it now and it reminds me of exactly how I felt. The treatment was finished and I was ecstatic to see Matt waiting outside to pick me up. We made it home where I continued to rest and I was even able to walk to the mailbox. I headed to bed early and waited to see what the next day would bring.

Although the treatment was uneventful it was only that way due to the wonderful nurses and staff at the Richard E. Winter Cancer Center. They did everything they could to make me comfortable. They worked together to make the IV as painless as possible because they knew that was what I dreaded most. I had opted out of a port, because the hospital is a place I did not care to be during the COVID19 pandemic. Their kindness and compassion would continue throughout my treatments and for that, I am forever grateful.

Words of Wisdom - Gratitude

May 3

Written By <u>Bridgette Akins</u>

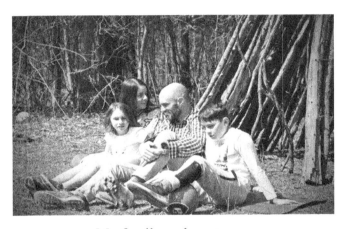

My family and our tepee.

Photo by Sarah Jacobs

Gratitude

"Breathing in, I calm body and mind. Breathing out, I smile. Dwelling in the present moment I know this is the only moment."
Thich Nhat Hanh

Happy May! Today's entry is on a simple but often overlooked topic, gratitude. Although during times such as these I find it easier to practice gratitude as I've been gifted with extra time for meditation and contemplation. Below are easy ways to practice gratitude. Practicing gratitude not only benefits those that we are grateful for but it also enriches our own life with joy and contentment.

Breathe - Last week I shared the importance of focused breathing and it is back again this week. We all know the physical importance of breathing but the next time you take in a breath be mindful. Mindful of the plants that produce the oxygen you breathe in and the carbon dioxide you breathe out that is absorbed by plant life. Be mindful and just say thank you.

Music - Find a song that speaks to you and listen or sing with mindfulness and passion. Really connect with the notes and words.

Acknowledge Others - Make a list of three people for whom you are grateful. Then, commit to acknowledging each of these people this week. Maybe it is a letter, a thank you or a thoughtful gift. It may be someone with whom you are really close or someone like a postal worker or acquaintance.

However, you choose to show gratitude just choose to do it boldly and whole heartedly.

Love and Laughter,
Bridgette

Words of Wellness - Acknowledging a Higher Power

For me it is my faith in God. I can see his grace in all of creation. I like to spend time outdoors admiring his beautiful creation. Nature is a great reminder of how much thought, care and love He puts into the world and if He provides for the lilies and the sparrows, He will also provide for me.

Spend time outside today.

Find a quiet spot and observe the natural elements that surround you.

Consider that there is something greater than yourself and try to connect to that greater power.

Use the space below to draw what you see and jot down thoughts about the greater power you connect with or possibilities of something greater that you wish to explore.

Acknowledging Others

When we think of natural wonders, we often overlook one of the most amazing wonders, people. So today I challenge you to really notice the people around you.

Begin by noticing the people you come in contact with today. Whether in passing or those that you spend time with in conversation.

Notice the beauty of their differences, their similarities, their words and their actions.

Choose three people to acknowledge. Maybe you give a stranger a compliment, say thank you to someone who supports you or pay it forward as an act of giving.

The world is beautiful and one of the reasons why is the people that live in it. Let us choose to notice and acknowledge all people.

Chapter Four: MoFa-What Are You Fighting For?

"Sometimes we're tested not to show our weaknesses but to discover our strengths."

Unknown

Since my surgery I had connected with a friend of a friend that was fighting her own battle against breast cancer and she told me if I only did one thing I should walk every day and I took that to heart. So, even if only to the mailbox I was going to try and walk every day. The fresh air always gave me a jolt of energy.

I was so excited about the way I had felt the initial days after my first treatment. Then things changed. I didn't sleep well through the night but I was able to sleep in. I was more tired than the day before but other than that I was only feeling achy kind of like thc flu. That was until the evening. This is when I had my first glimpse of what the side effects of chemo could be. I developed a pain that was like nothing I had ever felt. I cried from physical pain and emotional exhaustion. It was a harsh realization that this is chemo, this is cancer and this is my reality. I made it through the night with pain in my bones, joints and places I didn't even know could have pain. I was so thankful to have a heated blanket and wake to the following verse in my devotion.

"Come to me, all who are weary and burdened and
I will give you rest. "
Matthew 11:28

There had been so many changes in the last couple of months and we still weren't living at home. It was also a time of many difficult conversations. We had explained to the kids that I had cancer, the doctors had removed it during surgery and none was left but I had to have medicine as a precautionary measure.

The next days were great days and my daughter, Eva, reached a childhood milestone of riding her bike. An accomplishment that gave her so much pride especially during these crazy times. Just as it made her proud, it made this mommy proud as well. Unfortunately, over the next couple of days, I started having abdominal pain. I remembered the nurse saying when in doubt call and so I did. Blood work, x-ray, and cat scan were ordered and all came back normal. After an agonizing bowel movement, days later, the pain subsided and I focused on what the next treatment would bring.

I think I really found my strength before I even realized it. I knew I needed to prioritize myself and really embark on the journey of self-care. As a mom, wife, teacher and health coach, it was really hard for me to take steps in caring for myself when I had so many other people counting on me. But that was just it. They were counting on me. I have an extremely supportive family, wonderful support system, but how could I be there for them without being there for myself first? I had to realize that in order to get better, in order to be there for those that were counting on me, I had to find my MoFa: my motivating factor. I was going through chemo, recovering from surgery, trying to get myself through all of the things that happened in what seemed like the blink of an eye, and I realized how much I needed help. I needed to embrace the difficulty, embrace the pain, embrace the changes, and accept that it was going to lead to something beautiful.

Being a teacher and health coach, I find comfort in creating themes and plans so going into my second treatment I decided to create a theme for each of my chemo sessions. The theme for my second treatment was You Are My Sunshine. I had a soft, yellow blanket and a wore a yellow shirt. The theme and these items helped shift my mindset to one of light, hope and positivity. Little did I know this theme was going to come to life. As I went in, I was surprised to find that I would be joined by my Aunt Shannon who was also receiving treatment, and that wasn't the end of the surprise. You can read about the rest of the surprise in Words of Wisdom.

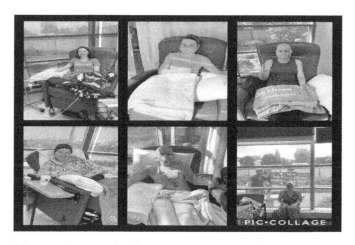

Photos from each of my 6 treatments. These photos
can be seen in color at www.bridgetteakins.com.

Words of Wisdom - MoFa - What Are You Fighting For?

May 13

Written By <u>Bridgette Akins</u>

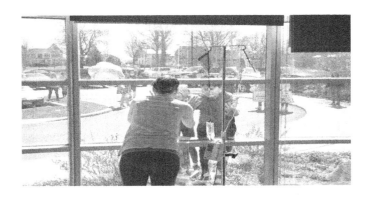

My Motivating Factor

You Are My Sunshine!

Yesterday was one of the most amazing days of my life. It was a perfect reminder of what I'm fighting for, my motivating factor (MoFa), my faith and my family. Tuesday was my second chemo treatment, which I themed 'You Are My Sunshine'. Due to COVID-19 I am accustomed to doing all things cancer related alone but this time was different. Our Aunt Shannon had her infusion changed to the same time as mine and requested that we be next to each other. The nurses were so kind to accommodate her request. It was so great to have someone to chat with and share stories. I'm usually there five and a half hours and just doze on and off. Little did I know that this wasn't all Shannon had planned. She had the nurses set our chairs facing the parking lot because she organized a family car parade to encourage me. My husband, kids and mother in law were first in line and I thought it was just them. My heart was so happy and I was so excited that I spilled my drink everywhere. Then I realized that there were many more cars with signs, balloons and well wishes. I'm not usually someone that cries but my heart was overflowing with love and my eyes with tears of joy. I can't put into words how special I felt. And at that moment everything was peaceful and everything was clear. These people were my MoFA. I was fighting for my kids, my husband, all my relationships and I am able to do this through my faith. That is what gives me a firm foundation and gives me strength beyond measure.

Today I challenge you to answer the questions: What is your MoFa? What are you fighting for?

Words of Wellness – Motivating Factor

In today's Words of Wellness, we focus on discovering your own motivating factor (MoFa), and developing anchors that will remind you of that MoFa and its importance.

MoFa – Motivating Factor

What are the factors in your life that will motivate and push you to fight, succeed and conquer even when things get tough or seem dire?

Make a list of these factors below. Following each factor describe why it motivates you.

Once the list is complete choose which will be your MoFa. It is okay to have more than one but you don't want to have so many that they lose their meaning and just become clutter.

Anchors

Now that you have discovered your MoFa it is time

to create anchors. Anchors are things in your physical environment that will remind you of your MoFa. Whatever you are facing there will inevitably be times of doubt, fear, sadness and setbacks. It is during these times that your anchors will remind you of your MoFa and positive thoughts and feelings.

You will create an anchor for each of your five senses. Choose one of your senses to begin.

Once you have chosen a sense think of an anchor to attach to that sense. This should be something that you see or do often. Examples of my anchors are listed below.

Complete an anchor for each of your senses.
Whenever you feel down, defeated or just need a pick me up think of your anchors and the MoFa they support.

Bridgette's Anchors
Sight – wedding band
Sound – Music - More Than Anything by Natalie

Grant

Taste – Chocolate Milkshake/Ice Cream

Smell – Fresh Air

Touch – Holding the hand of my husband and children

My Anchors

Sight –

Sound -

Taste –

Smell –

Touch -

Chapter Five: Stay Positive

"You are braver than you believe, stronger than you seem and smarter than you think." Christopher Robin

In the fifth week post-surgery, the chemo came into play. After the first round, it just crushed me physically, actually, in a lot of ways. I had really intense bone pain that lasted for five days and then things started happening and we knew I was going to lose my hair. We had already had the initial conversation with our children but it was time for more details. My husband and I had both said it, "You know, we've got to tell the kids." and the time had come to do just that. It was really just like, "Mom had cancer, and they got it all but this was what we have to do. This medicine is called chemo and it's going to make mommy lose her hair and that's what you're going to notice." Very quickly after this, I really started shedding hair, and so we cut my hair for the first time. An hour later and fourteen inches gone, I was sporting a pixie cut.

It wasn't long after my second treatment that my hair really started to fall out. Handfuls of hair would come out at a time and hair was all over everything from shirts to towels and even my eye mask. I went for my second haircut and this time we used just the clippers. Over the next couple of days, the pain set in once again. I had received a different pain medicine after this treatment but it didn't help nearly as much as I had hoped. It was during these times that it was hard to keep my spirits up. I just wanted the pain to go away and for this to all be over. I longed to be strong and healthy again. But, through it all, I knew God was in control and that he would bring me through in some way. I received a care package from dear friends and it couldn't have come at a better time as the weekend was tough not just physically but also mentally and emotionally. So many times, throughout my journey I was given strength through words of encouragement, cards, gifts and prayers. A strong support system made this journey much more bearable and much less lonely. It was only a few days after my second hair cut that it was time. Time to shave my head. My scalp was so itchy and hair was falling out at an alarming and gross rate. Matt and our son, Jack, both took turns with the clippers. Eva who has struggled most with the changing of my hair hid in the camper and couldn't bear to watch. It was an emotional process and I definitely cried but I knew it was time. The hardest was catching a glimpse of my reflection in the bumper of the camper and not recognizing myself. It was like seeing a stranger and that is when the tears came. However, once the shave was done, I was able to shower and then really look at my face in the mirror. I could tell it looked better than the patchy thinning hair that was there moments before. I also really noticed my eyes, my skin tone and my smile and I thought my face was beautiful!

Times like this were a little emotional because no matter how good I felt some days there were constant reminders that I wasn't healthy such as a bald head, nausea or just feeling bad out of the blue. One positive about the bad days was that they truly made me appreciate the good ones.

A photo timeline from long hair to no hair.
Color photos can be found at
www.bridgetteakins.com.

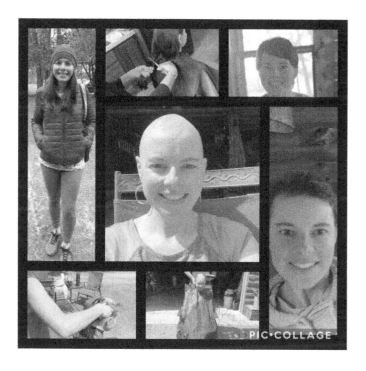

Words of Wisdom - Stay Positive

May 28

Written By <u>Bridgette Akins</u>

Two words that are simple in meaning but powerful when put into practice. However, in our most challenging times in life, it is often hard to put these words into action. When it seems like our circumstances are ever-changing or never changing, when fear and failure seem more prevalent than joy and success staying positive becomes quite the task.

As someone who prides herself on being positive and strong, this journey is testing my ability to be just that. It was the week after my 2nd treatment that I really felt the struggle of staying positive. The bone pain had set in around day three and was still hanging out at day six. The treatment before I experienced the same pain but by day six it had subsided to aches, not pain. So I fully expected my body to stay on that schedule. To say that I was disappointed about the extra day of pain is an understatement. This is when I felt my positivity really being tested. I soaked in a hot bath, listened to my fight song, prayed (an odd place for worship but it's my place these days) and wondered what to do next.

As I relaxed I embraced the pain and all the emotions that came with it. It was during this time that the phrase Stay Positive kept surfacing in my thoughts. It was my Aha moment. For many years I have set goals and made vision boards to help me achieve those goals and now should be no different. My goals are usually more numerous and a little more complex but I knew in this time my goal was simple Stay Positive (although I haven't yet made a cancer vision board). I can't control the way the chemo treatments affect my body but I can control where I let my thoughts wander. I will continue to acknowledge and embrace the pain but overall I will fight to stay strong and positive.

Many of us are facing our own life battle during this

time. I wholeheartedly believe that whatever your journey that this too shall pass for all of us. As we navigate life I challenge you to embrace what you can, let go of what doesn't serve you and above all STAY POSITIVE.

Love and Laughter,
Bridgette

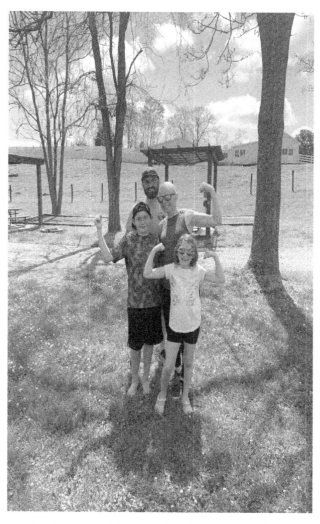

Photo taken on Virginia camping trip with my parents and niece.

Words of Wellness - Goals

It is now time for you to set your goal or goals for this challenge. You may choose one goal or multiple goals. As stated above my goal was Stay Positive. Below are some tips for creating your goal(s).

Goals

Be positive. State what you want not what you don't want.

Make sure this is a goal centered around you.
Create a description of how you will know that you have met this goal. What will it look and/or feel like?

Keep it simple yet powerful and meaningful. You don't want to create a goal so complex that it is unattainable.

Choose a date or time frame in which to accomplish

the goal. It is okay if the timeframe spans your entire treatment or journey.

Support System

After creating your goal make a list of those people in your life that can help you achieve that goal. These people will become your support system and will be crucial during your journey with this challenge.

Chapter Six: Expect the Unexpected

"The Lord goes before you and will be with you. He will never leave or forsake you. Therefore, do not be afraid, do not be discouraged."

Deuteronomy 3:18

For anyone that has tackled cancer and its treatment you know the importance of the phrase "Expect the Unexpected." Just as you feel you have one thing under control another thing changes. I was feeling pretty good and Matt and I were headed to the hospital for my scheduled blood work prior to the third chemo treatment. It went well with no pain and we headed home to enjoy the day. Much to my surprise, I received a call that afternoon that I would not be able to receive my treatment the next day due to my white blood count being too low.

I took it pretty hard. We scheduled a camping trip for the following week and I had mapped out dates for all of my treatments. This allowed me to feel like I had some control but alas that wasn't the case. I cried and shared the news with Matt. It was disappointing and pushed all of my treatments a week but in the end, there was nothing I could do. I just had to wait until my blood count came up on its own. We scheduled blood work for the following Monday and possible treatment for Tuesday. If all went well, we would still be able to make it to the campground Tuesday night. Being that emotional always made me tired but I was prayerful and optimistic that my body was going to get stronger and things would get back on track.

During all of this uncertainty, I wasn't the only one in the family dealing with the unexpected. Jack, whose birthday is in December, decided to postpone his celebration last year so that he could do something with his friends when the weather was warmer. Unfortunately, the pandemic and cancer weren't going to let that happen. Even though he couldn't be with his friends we wanted to find a way to celebrate and bring some normalcy back to our lives and the family was there to help. His Aunt Brigid and cousin Maddy spent the day with him playing soccer, making a giant no-bake cookie and letting him have soda. We had sloppy joes and lobster tails for dinner and brownies, ice cream and the giant no-bake for dessert. The candles were relighting which made for a comical moment. We wrapped up the evening with a llama piñata and everyone taking a turn until it finally burst open sending goodies everywhere. Eva even spent her own money to buy Jack a football and table football game. Both of which he loves to play with his dad. Although these things may seem mundane, they were exactly what he and all of us needed. Especially since we would soon have another unexpected event.

Eva's change was unfortunately not a welcome one. The night before my fourth treatment she knocked out her front tooth while riding her bike. And yes, it was a permanent tooth. It was a scary situation but from putting the tooth into milk to calling ahead to the ER our family worked together to give us the best chance in saving Eva's tooth. After all of this work we were turned away at the first emergency room. They claimed no doctor could help with the tooth. I pride myself in being calm but as I looked at my crying, toothless, bleeding daughter I unleashed the wrath of a mother who had just been denied treatment of her child. After being turned away by one emergency room we arrived at another and the ER doctor, oral surgeon, myself and Matt worked to secure the tooth. She was strong and courageous through it all. The next days were filled with a swollen sore lip and anxiety about being sedated for the root canal that would need to be done.

All of the uncertainty and changes were difficult but one was more so than all the others. A challenge that is common but often not talked about... connection and intimacy.

With everything going on Matt and I felt like we rarely had time to sit and chat by ourselves let alone be intimate. Our lives had been upended and we hadn't been home in three months. We finally found a spot in the schedule where we could have some alone time and yes, we had to schedule the time by ourselves. So, for others that feel the strain of not having time with your spouse or partner, schedule it in just like any other very important appointment and you will make it happen. Even if it is only 15 minutes here or there the connection is worth it. Matt and I were able to have lunch and just chat about everything. It was so uplifting to be able to connect with this person that is my rock whom I saw every day but, in the craziness, didn't always connect.

Challenge one was finding time to truly connect and we had conquered that challenge. The next was much more difficult. We were a married couple who before all of this had a healthy and amazing love life but all that had changed. From the beginning, all of this just killed any kind of intimacy we had beforehand, and so that was really hard. I think that was one of the hardest parts. Having a full hysterectomy had changed my body and the chemo was doing the same. The physical pain is difficult of course, but then feeling like you've changed, thinking that nothing was going to be the way that it was. That was devastating.

Thankfully, I have an amazing and supportive husband who in no way pushed that part of our marriage during this journey. He kissed me, told me I was beautiful and reminded me that this was an amazing part of our marriage but it wasn't the only part of our marriage. He was still so in love with me and for now our intimacy would look different. We could hold each other, kiss and hug each other, hold hands and shower each other with words of affection. I cannot express how amazing it is to have a strong marriage and a strong husband whose love is truly unconditional.

Like everyone else, we had been quarantined for the last nine weeks but unlike most, we hadn't been home either. Cancer is not only difficult on the person diagnosed but also their family, friends and community. I hadn't seen my parents since Christmas and they were anxious to see their baby girl. Being apart during this time was not easy. We were all excited to have the opportunity to meet up for Memorial Day weekend in Virginia and with no travel restrictions in place we were going to be able to do just that. Of course, there were some lingering side effects of fatigue and nausea but luckily medicine and a chocolate milkshake helped. We were able to play cards and games, wade in the creek, cook over the fire and make ice cream sundaes. The time to visit was therapeutic for all and Jack and Eva were ecstatic to receive gifts from their mamaw and papaw.

Again, no matter how good I felt some days the ugly side effects always seemed to be right around the corner. I didn't want my parents to see me sick. They were worried enough and I wanted their memories of this weekend to be of me happy, full of life and positivity. For the most part, I was able to accomplish just that. Through all of the unexpected, I sometimes held in the emotions and sometimes I could not. In summary, it was a crazy ride!

Words of Wisdom – Strong and Still

Jun 15

Written By <u>Bridgette Akins</u>

"I want to be a powerful force of gentle peace in a world that needs you."
Kathi Lipp - Proverbs 31 Devotional"

Throughout this journey many people have told me that I am strong and I do believe that. However, there have been times in the last few months that I have wondered if I really am as strong as they think I am. It was during these times that I rediscovered some life truths that I also find applicable to the many crises that face our nation.

You can be Strong and Still Cry.
You can be Strong and Still be Kind.
You can be Strong and Still feel Alone.

You can be Strong and Still be Humble.

You can be Strong and Still feel Anger.

You can be Strong and Still be Peaceful.

This is a pivotal time to listen to our fellow Americans that are being and have been persecuted. It's time to learn how we can be active participants in the fight against racism and inequality. Just like with cancer and chemotherapy it might get uncomfortable even painful but we need to understand what is unfolding in our nation. It's time we witness and internalize all that is happening and let these events uncover emotions. We should embrace these emotions, contemplate and act. Let these feelings be a light to join with others and fight for true equality, justice and freedom for all. Be strong for change and love not for violence and hate.

Be Strong and Courageous - Joshua 1:9
Be Still and Know - Psalm 46:10

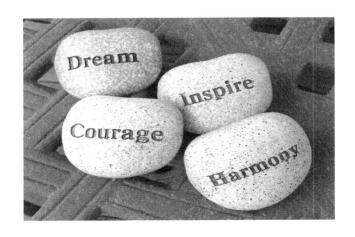

Words of Wellness - "I Am" Statements

Grab a pen and paper.

Find a quiet spot and set a timer for 5 minutes.

Sit tall, notice your breath and relax any tension in your body.

Recall the challenge you are currently facing and think of what it will take for you to conquer this challenge.

Write down as many "I Am" statements that come to mind.

After the 5 minutes read your list and circle 3 statements.

Repeat your "I Am" statements each day or when needed.

Example "I Am" Statements

I am an overcomer.

I am courageous.

I am willing to invest in me.

I am beautiful.

I am able.

Chapter Seven: One Step at A Time

"Year's end is neither an end nor a beginning but a
going on with all the wisdom that experience can
instill in us."
Hal Borland

After feeling overwhelmed by the unexpected it was going to be nice to escape to the Adirondacks for the week before heading back to Albany. We were all looking forward to going home in June after being away for 13 weeks. When talking to someone at the cancer center about traveling home it sounded so surreal and made me a little emotional. I was going home if only for a little over a week but first Lake Placid. Matt and I have always labeled Lake Placid as our special place and we cherish any time that we can spend there. We were excited to have this time with our kids and just unplug.

Matt and the kids drove the RV to pick me up from

my treatment and we made it to the campground for dinner. The next several days were amazing as I only experienced minimal pain and being in the mountains was so calming. Matt made meals, washed dishes and entertained the kids so I could rest. I was able to go on a short walk with the kids the first day but fatigue was more intense this time. While I rested Matt and the kids set out on their own adventure; a bike, hike, swim. They biked six miles, hiked three and did a little wading, swimming in the river. I was so proud of the kids and their perseverance and ability to get along. Over the next few days, I felt amazing compared to the way I felt after previous treatments. These days were usually riddled with pain but not this time and I was going to take advantage of it. Family members joined us at the campground and we were able to do a hike together and although I wasn't able to make it as far as I'd hoped I was so proud of myself for getting out and trying. The kids played and we were able to chat as adults. It really was ideal.

As ideal as it was, we were ready to head home. We

made our trip back to Albany eventful, stopping at a few special places including Adirondack Chocolates, the Keene Farmers Market and Fat Daddy's Hot Dog Stand. It is so important to take advantage of the time we have together and make each day as special as we can. After three hours we pulled into the driveway. It felt as if this was the first time pulling into a brand-new home and my eyes filled with tears of joy. The kids and I documented the moment with a picture on the front steps before we went inside. I spent time in each room of the house and sitting on the back porch taking it all in. I was happy to be home but my mind was racing with all of the organizing and redecorating that I was planning. There was something more that I was feeling I just hadn't figured it out yet.

Words of Wisdom – One Step

Jun 19

Written By <u>Bridgette Akins</u>

Sunday will mark one week since we returned home. We left in March for a long weekend and now three and a half months later we finally made it back. Needless to say, a lot has happened in our lives, in your life and in our nation. I've never stayed anywhere (except home) for more than a few weeks, six weeks at max and that was for a summer job during college . Being a way for several months I felt like home was somewhere else. Don't get me wrong I was in the best place possible. We were able to stay with my husband's parents in the beautiful north country of New York. Their love and support made the challenging circumstances not only doable but filled with love and joy.

However, as we started planning and packing to return it felt strange, and the first time I spoke about it to someone else I experienced a wave of different emotions. It all seemed surreal. I was teary eyed with excitement, anxiety, joy and sadness. As I continued to plan and pack, I spent time with my thoughts and realized all of the feelings were valid. They allowed me to appreciate all that had happened the last three months and look forward to all that was ahead. I was ready to go home.

As I stated in the introduction, we arrived home about a week ago. The kids and I took the picture below to mark this special moment. It felt like we were moving in for the first time. I took time to walk around outside and absorb all that I had missed. The beautiful maple in the front yard, the open and secluded back yard with a tree drooping with cherries. After a while I made my way inside to the place we live and call home. It was just as I had remembered but with a different feeling. As we unpacked the car and put everything inside, I began envisioning how I would redecorate and verbally listing all of the things I wanted to buy. I started a mental to do list of rooms and items to declutter and I was ready to get started on Monday. For those that know me this isn't really a new thing as I love to organize and declutter any given day but this was different. However, I didn't realize how different until we were winding down for the night. I begin to chat with my husband about getting rid of clothes and changing things when he asked me why.

It only took me a split second before my emotions overwhelmed me. I hadn't really taken the time to process being home and what that meant. Now that he had posed the simple question of why, I suddenly knew. This was my home and everything seemed the same except it wasn't. Before we left in March I was working, the kids were in school and we were free to rush along with our busy schedules. I was healthy, although not feeling well, and never dreamed of a cancer diagnosis. So, although home seemed the same, I knew deep down it would never be the same again. This was a scary thought accompanied by sadness and it also seemed to come out of nowhere.

I was so excited to be home so it was hard for me to understand how these emotions seemed to come from nowhere. For the first time I felt like I could get lost in those thoughts and emotions.

Luckily, I was able to sleep and although I can't say I felt completely relieved in the morning I was able to tell myself to take it one step at a time. For me the first step was to pray and stay positive. Then, I kept myself busy and started organizing which I find very therapeutic. All the while I reminded myself of my MoFa (motivating factor) which is all of those that love and support me and some that depend on me. There were many activities throughout the week that filled me with joy and brought happy tears. With each spark of happiness my feelings of sadness and despair were replaced with hope.

It's been almost a week, the house is organized and I am finally at a place where I can acknowledge and appreciate my "new" home. I know the process isn't complete but I know that I only have to take one step at a time. Sometimes the step may be forward and sometimes I may need to take a step back. Either way, I have a life to live and I plan to live it with love and laughter.

What has challenged you during this time of uncertainty and quarantine?
What is the first step you can take to overcome this challenge?

As always,
Love and Laughter,
Bridgette

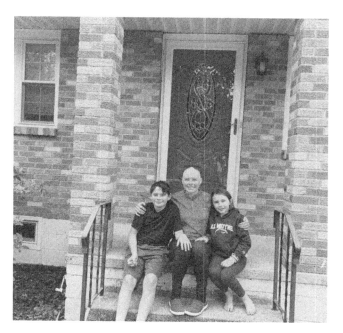

Home Sweet Home

Words of Wellness – Nourishment Menu

Stressors/Relaxers

Take 2-3 minutes and think of the different things that cause you stress and those that help you to relax. Use the lines below to write down your top three stressors and top three relaxers.

Top 3 Stressors   Top 3 Relaxers

_____   _____

_____   _____

_____   _____

Nourishment Menu

Next, you are going to create a nourishment menu. This is a menu full of choices that allow you to relax or experience pleasure. Some things on my nourishment menu are hot baths, massage, yoga, flowers and chocolate. Have fun creating your own menu!

My Nourishment Menu

_____

_____

_____

_____

_____

_____

_____

_____

_____

_____

_____

_____

_____

_____

_____

_____

_____

_____

Chapter Eight: Faith, Hope, Love

"And now these three remain: faith, hope and love.
But the greatest of these is love."
1 Corinthians 13:13

After settling in at home and acknowledging my different thoughts and emotions life seemed to take on some resemblance of normalcy. Although I knew this was short-lived as my next treatment was in a couple of weeks. We enjoyed the time at home as a family doing many of the things we had missed while being away. We went to the farmers market and ate at one of our favorite restaurants, outdoors of course. We were able to celebrate Father's Day and end of school parades. We were also able to visit with a couple of friends which gave us all a huge emotional boost. We grilled out and had lots of s'mores over the fire. During this time, I was also able to reflect and meditate on my journey thus far. The three components that were constant throughout my journey were faith, hope and love.

Faith

From day one I leaned on my faith in God to get me through every day, every ache, every success and every setback. Sometimes it was through my daily devotion, other times it was through worship music or a walk outside. No matter how important or how insignificant I thought something was I would pray about it. This allowed me to let it go and take a sigh of relief. Now, it wasn't always easy to let it go and I didn't always do it right away. Sometimes I prayed the same prayer over and over. Sometimes I would fixate on a problem or how awful I felt but there always came a time that I handed it over to God and when I made that choice my heart, mind and body felt at peace.

Hope

I mentioned my faith above and that obviously gave me hope but there were other places where I saw hope. Every time I looked at my husband and saw the amount of work and love he put into our family I saw hope. Hope that I would be cancer free but if not, I knew we would be ok. When I saw my children playing or smiling up at me while we snuggled, I saw hope. Hope that despite the circumstances they were experiencing joy and love. When I walked outside and felt the sun and wind on my skin, saw the beautiful colors of flowers and trees and heard the sounds of animals I saw hope. Hope that the creator of all things would nurture me just as he was nurturing these things.

Love

Just as the verse in Corinthians states the greatest of these things is love. I could not have made it through my journey without love. The love of my husband, Matt, who while working took over most of the family chores and responsibilities so I could focus on my treatments. He constantly showered me with kind words and gestures. My children, Jack and Eva, who despite all the changes in their lives, found ways to care for me with hugs, kisses, snuggles, helping out with chores and reassuring me that it was all going to be ok and that they still loved me even without hair.

My in-laws, Jane and Gordie Akins, opened their home for us to live in for six months and helped us keep up with the everyday like laundry and meals. The love of my parents, Teresa and Dickie Lay, almost 1,000 miles away, who constantly checked in and sent me sweet gifts in the mail. The love of family, friends and strangers was remarkable. There were so many times that I would have a rough day or feel emotional and that very day I would receive a card, text or gift from someone. These things picked me up and gave me the motivation at just the right time. Prayers of love were lifted from all parts of the world and the power of those prayers helped me fight even the toughest days. As you read today's Words of Wisdom it is just one example of seeing faith, hope and love in the everyday things.

Words of Wisdom – Faith, Hope, Love

Jul 13

Written By <u>Bridgette Akins</u>

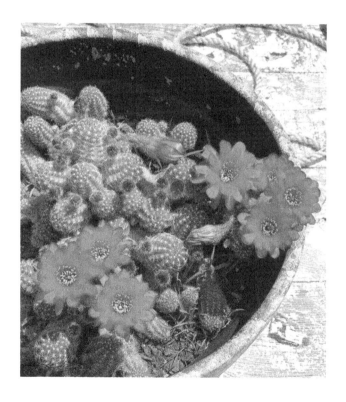

And now these three remain: faith, hope and love.

But the greatest of these is love.

1 Corinthians 13:13

A verse of simple words yet filled with power. Words I have always found vital but never more so than now. The picture above isn't one of photographic perfection yet it is one of perfection just the same. My son took this picture of his flowering cactus. A cactus that embodies faith, hope and love. As many know the last few months have been filled with unexpected adventures and change for us. At the top of the list includes corona-virus, my diagnosis with ovarian cancer and our quarantine away from home for three months. It was during this time away that the cactus became so important.

As my husband and son prepared to make a quick trip home to gather some necessary items, we made a list of what we would need and want. The usual items were first on the list, clothes, medicine, outdoor gear and then we moved to wants. Being away from home for months at a time can be hard on anyone but with so much change I was worried most about my children. Don't get me wrong they loved being with their grandparents and cousins but it was a lot to take in. So, as we continued the list I wasn't surprised that stuffed animals, blankets, and soccer stuff made the cut. I was however surprised at the request for the cactus.

A little background on the cactus. We have had said cactus for about five years and it lives in a beautiful pot decorated with fingerprints from my daughter and her friends in North Carolina. It is beautiful but heavy. The pot and cactus probably weigh twenty-five pounds not to mention it isn't easy to transport four hours in a car. I knew this wasn't going to make the cut. As we discussed it with my son his sincerity and passion were abundant. He wanted to bring the cactus, because he was afraid he was going to miss it blooming. That might not seem like a big deal but we knew from experience that it usually only bloomed once or twice during the summer and the rest of the year it was just a green cactus. As we continued the discussion, I realized that the cactus was a symbol of hope and normalcy for him. He had faith that in a time so different that the cactus was going to bloom just the same and he truly loved it.

We weren't able to bring the cactus but we talked about it often and I prayed that it would not only survive until we got home but that he wouldn't miss it bloom. After three months we came home to a still living cactus but no idea if it had reached the blooming point. A few days later we noticed the buds and shortly after we were able to watch them bloom. A moment that meant so much. A moment that had to be captured in a photo. In anything but an ordinary year we also got an extraordinary surprise. The cactus has had several blooms since the first ones died. Something we have never seen.

The cactus became a symbol of faith, hope and love. Things we can all strive to show a little more. Just as faith helped him believe that the cactus was going to be okay, coupled with hope that he wouldn't miss the flowers and love for all that this plant represented it also became a symbol for me.

Our faith in God, ourselves and others should be unwavering even if we can't see the changes we long to see. Hope is always available even when conditions aren't ideal or even treacherous. Love is patient and love is kind. Love is most important of the three. Like a prickly cactus so many are waiting to be patiently loved so that they can bloom into the best version of themselves and show the world the beauty that is deep inside.

Where do your faith and hope come from?

What can you do today or this week to show others that they are loved?

How can you show self-love?

Love and Laughter,

Bridgette

Words of Wellness – Empowering Lessons

WOW Moments

What WOW moments or empowering lessons have you learned throughout this challenge?

Write down three WOW moments or empowering lessons that you have learned from your journey.

I learned

_____

_____

I learned

_____

_____

I learned

_____

_____

Chapter Nine: The Future Never Looked So Good!

"I love who I have been but I really love who I am becoming."

Dulce Ruby

There's a reason people battling cancer get depressed because you're not in control of your body any longer and you can't stop the changes from happening. The thing is, you still have the real world to contend with. Things like scheduling doctor appointments, paying for treatments and surgery, and a thousand other things. If you can find clarity and positivity, and make sure you have a good support system, those mundane things become so much less stressful. Sitting in your feelings of being overwhelmed, depressed, and feeling self-conscious about everything that's going on, it doesn't serve you. Increased anxiety and worry, low self-esteem, living in fear, you kind of fall into having a journey that controls you instead of the other way around. When this happens remember your Mofa? The motivating factor. Maybe yours is a mantra, maybe it's the goal of overcoming, and for me, it was being positive.

As my journey continued, my last treatment approached. I was excited and emotional. I couldn't believe the final treatment was here. As always Matt drove me to my treatment but today, he had a surprise. Our moms had coordinated with family and friends to have cards and gifts for me to open for my last day of chemo (see pics below). I was overwhelmed with the outpouring of love from all over the world. Aunt Shannon scheduled her infusion to coincide with mine so once again I wouldn't have to be alone. I was excited to ring the bell at the conclusion of my treatment but was also sad that Matt and the kids wouldn't be able to join me. As I exited the restroom and headed to ring the bell, I was surprised not only by the nurses singing to me but to see Matt, Jack and Eva singing along as well. I was the only patient remaining and they checked them all before allowing them to enter. It was so special to share this with them as we were all on this cancer journey together.

As excited as I was to complete treatment, I knew there were still side effects to come and that I had one more IV for my cat scan and one more follow up with Dr. A. The side effects came as did the cat scan and follow up doctor's visit. It was here that Dr. A gave me the great news that according to the scan and blood test I was cancer free. After conversation and many questions, it was time for me to leave. As I walked out of the cancer center, I knew that I was done that I had survived this journey. Matt and Jack were waiting for me and as soon as I headed toward the car, I began to get teary eyed. It wasn't until I was able to hug Matt that I broke down with tears of joy and relief. This was a feeling like I had never felt before and for the first time since surgery and diagnosis, I had been able to let go of everything. We were both so happy and relieved and we continued to embrace while we both cried. Jack's support and compassion were so sweet. This was by far one of the most amazing moments of my life.

We headed home for good and I have spent each day trying to figure out my new normal. Every day is different and I am learning to roll with it. Being patient is perhaps the most difficult new challenge. I want to have energy and go back to doing all the things I had done before my diagnosis but it isn't that easy.

My last treatment was the end of one chapter but the beginning of several more. I welcome every day with prayer, love and laughter and I wish the same for you!

Words of Wisdom – Faith Over Fear

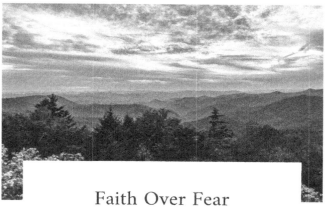

Faith Over Fear

Throughout my journey with cancer I set a
goal to stay positive. For the most part I was
able to do just that and put faith over fear. I
knew the importance of that statement
during my treatments but I didn't realize
how much I would lean on it throughout my
recovery.

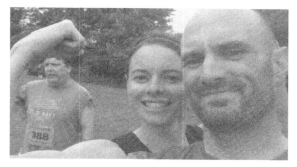

Faith Over Fear

As the days have passed since my final treatment the thing I have struggled with most is patience. Specifically, patience with myself. I want so much to feel myself again but lingering side effects have made that a challenge. The pictures on the cover remind me of the physical strength I once had and hope to gain again soon. The mountains remind me that God is with me when I am on top and also when I am walking in a valley. As I continue this journey of joy and tears my song will be that of faith over fear!

Love and Laughter,

Bridgette

Words of Wellness – Future Goals

Future Goals

No matter where you are in this challenging journey it is time to look to the future. Maybe the future is this month, this year or this lifetime. No matter when it is, now is the time to look to it with hope and positivity.

Use the space below to list things you'd like to complete in the future. Remember the future can be any time frame, this month, this year or this lifetime.

You may choose to use the following prompts to help you organize your thoughts.

I want to focus on _____.

Why is that important?

Are there any habits/strategies that I can use to support this focus or will I need outside support?

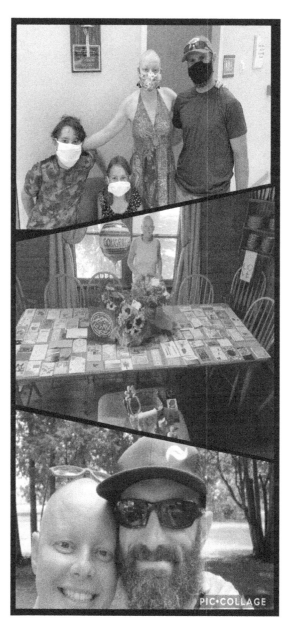

We did it!

Chapter Ten: Words of Warriors

"Live as if you were to die tomorrow, learn as if you were to live forever."
Gandhi

If you're faced with a difficulty that feels insurmountable, there are so many different methods you could use to overcome. What worked for me, what made me successful in my journey is finding my MoFa. The first step is to figure out why you're doing this. Even if it's not cancer, why are you fighting to get through this situation? What is your motivating factor or MoFa?

Next, choose your goal or mantra. Mine was, "Be positive."

Then, choose that thing that's going to anchor you to it, mine was a song. Finally, commit to the "I am" statements. Come up with at least one statement, "I am strong." "I am a survivor.' to say, believe and live out.

This is a journey of clarity, confidence, peace, and positivity. When you're enduring some of the hardest things in your life, when things have changed your life, how can you be true to yourself? Or how can you find the person you've wanted to be and have never been able to feel comfortable with?

How can you find the clarity in what you really want out of this journey and out of your life? How can you find the peace in order to let you really accept and really engage and embrace the process? How do you find the confidence to get you through the worst and the best times? And how do you stay positive? What are simple things that you can do to remind yourself that you don't have rainbows unless you have rain? And what are the simple things you can do to make this your journey? Remember, you define your journey, don't let the journey define you.

It is going to be hard. And you can do it, you're strong. Prioritize yourself, practice self-care, this is about you. You're going to take care of your kids, you're going to make time for your husband and your relationships. But it's going to look different and that's okay.

Always remember to ask for help and to give yourself grace. It is temporary. Even if your diagnosis was not like mine, if your diagnosis is that of stage 3, stage 4 and you have a year of chemo, the day is temporary. If you're trying to overcome an abusive situation, if you're trying to regain strength in yourself and in your life, if you're struggling in any way, remember, it is temporary.

Throughout this book we have focused on many WOWs. Every chapter brought new Words of Wisdom and Words of Wellness. You were also given the opportunity to record some of your own WOW moments. For the final WOW I thought it fitting that you document your story as a warrior. This is your opportunity to share how you were able to fight and overcome.

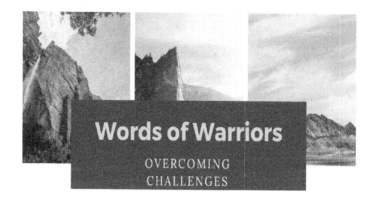

Words of Warriors

OVERCOMING
CHALLENGES

Throughout life's challenges there are highs (mountains), lows (valleys) and moments that inspire us to look toward the future (horizon). Below we meet warriors, those that have faced and overcome life challenges, and their WOW moments along the way.

Warrior Name:

My Journey

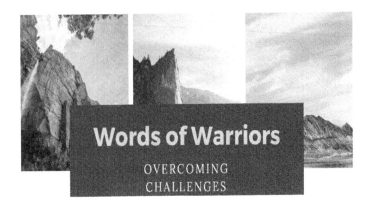

Words of Warriors

OVERCOMING CHALLENGES

Throughout life's challenges there are highs (mountains), lows (valleys) and moments that inspire us to look toward the future (horizon). Below we meet warriors, those that have faced and overcome life challenges, and learn how they have navigated life's journey.

Mountain

Valley

Horizon

Chapter Eleven: What's Next

"Each person holds so much power within themselves that needs to be let out. Sometimes they just need a little nudge, a little direction, a little support, a little coaching, and the greatest things can happen."
Pete Carroll

Are you ready to conquer your challenge but not sure where to start? Would you like to take a deeper dive into defining your journey?

Visit my website, bridgetteakins.com/services to receive a free 15-minute Discover You Interview, as well as a free gift delivered to your inbox. Find me on Instagram and Facebook @healthcoachingbybridgette to continue following my journey, while connecting with others and learning to define your own journey

I look forward to joining you on your journey and guiding you to a place of clarity, confidence, peace and positivity. Together we will Rise Up!

Love and Laughter,
Bridgette

Acknowledgments

Thank you to:

My husband, Matt, who has challenged me to meet all of my dreams and has supported me with an unwavering love and strength.

My kids, Jack and Evangeline, for being flexible and loving mommy through all of the uncertainties of COVID19 and cancer.

My parents, Dickie and Teresa Lay, for their unconditional love and support and the sacrifices they have always made for me.

My in-laws, Gordie and Jane Akins, for supporting us during this cancer journey with love, support, housing, meals and entertainment.

All of my family and friends that reached out with prayers, kind words, gifts, donations and meals.

Christine Vaughan and Bethlehem Children's School staff and families for their unwavering love and support.

The amazing doctors, nurses and support staff who cared for me along the way with love, compassion, kindness and respect.

Kathleen Maxian and the Ovarian Cancer Project for information and conversation.

Kidd Marketing for helping the dream of this book become a reality.

Sable Trappenburg, socialandspice.com, for her design expertise on my logo and website.

Amber Johns, ajpstudios518, for photos that truly help me see my beauty and strength.

Sasha Lay for the beautiful nature photos that she graciously shares with me (see cover photo).

All of the above mentioned and countless others have showered me with prayers, love, grace and kindness. I couldn't have made it through my cancer journey without each of them. I am eternally grateful for their support.

Made in the USA
Coppell, TX
01 December 2020

42492003R00075